Table of Contents

INTRODUCTION

The keto diet is a diet that has low carbs, has high fat and adequate protein. This diet allows the body to burn or remove enough fats instead of carbohydrates. The fat burned out of the body in turn serves as a source of energy for the body. Keto diet can also turn fat into ketones and this takes place in the liver. The ketones formed definitely produces energy to the brain. Keto diet is just so filling and it makes one loose weight without even counting calories or tracking your food intake. Because it is a high fat and low carb diet, ketogenic diet is mostly used by doctors to control epilepsy seizures.

Easy and Delicious Keto Diets: Recipes, Preparations and Nutritional Content

Here are recipes and directions of delicious keto diets to keep you healthy and fit in all activities of your life.

Cauliflower fried rice

Servings: 5 servings

Ingredients
For fried rice

- 1 head of cauliflower (cut into • florets)
- 3 tablespoons of vegetable oil
- 1 bunch of scallions (thinly sliced)
- 4 cloves of garlic(minced)

- 1 tablespoon of minced freshginger 3 teaspoons sriracha
- 3 carrots, (peeled and diced)
- 3 stalks of celery (diced)
- 1 red ball pepper (diced)
- 1 cup of frozen peas
- 2 tablespoons of rice vinegar
- 4 tablespoons of soy sauce

For Garnish

- 2 tablespoon of vegetable oil
- 5 eggs
- 5 tablespoons of chopped fresh cilantro
- 1 teaspoon of salt
- Black pepper(freshly ground)
- 5 teaspoons sesame seeds
- 5 tablespoons of scallions (thinly sliced)

Instructions

To make the fried rice:

- ✓ In a food processor, pulse the ✓ cauliflower until it resembles rice, 2-5 minutes, set aside.
- ✓ Put the olive oil in a skillet and ✓ heat over medium heat.
- ✓ Add scallions, ginger and garlic and stir for 2 minutes Add carrots, pepper and celery and ✓ fry until vegetable becomes tender, 9-12 minutes.
- ✓ Add the cauliflower rice, fry until ✓ color changes to golden, 3-6minutes more.
- ✓ Then stir in the 5 frozen peas and toss well to combine
- ✓ Add rice vinegar, sriracha and soy sauce. Set aside.

To make garnishes:

- ✓ Put oil in a medium skillet and heat over medium high heat.
- ✓ Beat the eggs directly into the pan and cook until the whites are set but the yolks still remains runny, about 3-5 minutes.
- ✓ Season each with pepper and salt to taste,

To serve:

- ✓   Divide the cauliflower rice among 5 plates and top each with the fried egg.
- ✓   Garnish each plate with 1 tablespoon scallions, 1-tablespoon cilantro and 1-teaspoon sesame seeds.
- ✓   Serve and enjoy.

Nutritional content (per serving)
Fried rice

Calories-108 Fat-1g Carbohydrate -22g Sugar-9g Protein -8g Garnishes
Calories -183 Fat- 7g Carb -3g Sugar- 0g

KETO WEDGE SALAD

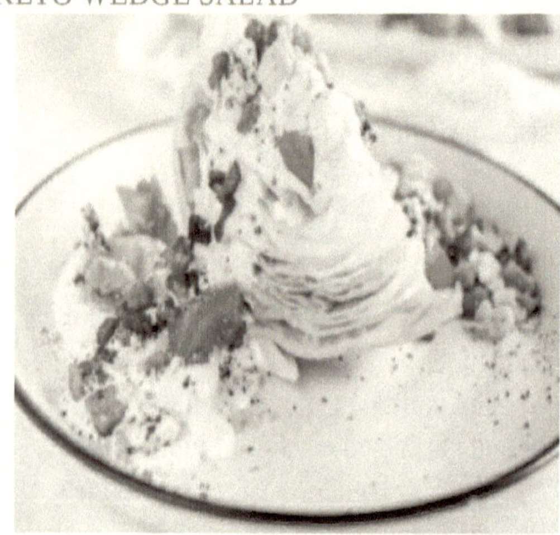

4 servings

Ingredients
Blue cheese dressing

- 2-tablespoons of heavy whipping cream
- One third cup of mayonnaise
- 2-ounces of blue cheese (crumbled)
- One quarter teaspoon of salt
- One quarter teaspoon of garlic powder
- One quarter cup of sour cream

- 1-tablespoon of lemon juice

Salad

- **4**-boiled eggs (chopped)
- 2-ounces of blue cheese (crumbled)
- Half head of iceberg lettuce
- 8-ounces of bacon (chopped)
- 1 tomato(chopped)

Instructions

✓ With the exception of the cheese, add all of the dressing ingredients in a mixing bowl. When all is well mixed, add the blue cheese and stir thoroughly. Depending on preference, a little water may be used to thin the mixture. Refrigerate until ready to eat.

✓ Over medium-high heat, cook the chopped bacon until it becomes crunchy in a large frying pan.

✓ Rinse and rinse the iceberg lettuce head in cold water. To dry the outside, use a clean towel.

✓ Break the lettuce head in half with a knife. To make four servings, split one half of the head into four wedges. To keep the lettuce fresh, leave the other half of the head alone.

✓ Place each wedge on a separate plate. On top, evenly distribute the bacon, blue cheese, chopped tomatoes, and egg. Dress the wedges all over with the dressing. Serve immediately.

KETO CHICKEN CURR BELL-PEPPER SANDWICH

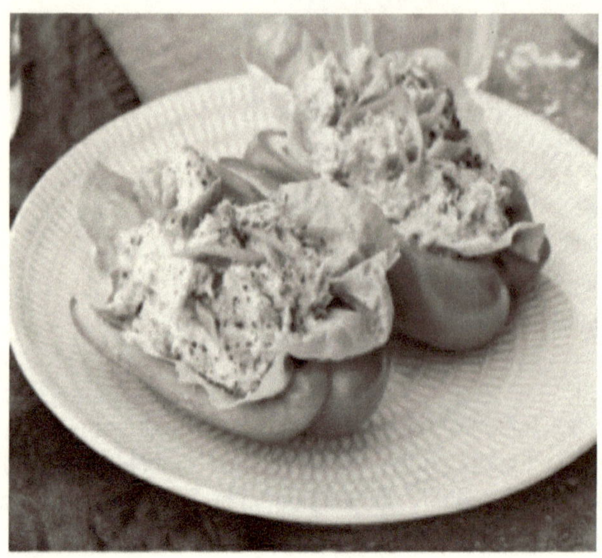

4 servings

Ingredients

- 2 red bell peppers
- 8-ounces of cooked chicken (cut into small pieces)
- 1 tablespoon of curry powder
- Salt and grounded black pepper
- One(1/2 oz.) scallion(finely sliced)
- 4 leaves of butter head lettuce
- Half cup of mayonnaise

Instructions

✓ Split the pepper seeds lengthwise to remove them and set them aside.

✓ In a mixing bowl, combine the chicken, mayonnaise, scallion, and curry; season with salt and pepper to taste.

✓ Keep a salad leaf on each half of a bell pepper, then spoon the chicken curry mixture into the pepper and top with scallions if desired.

TUNA STUFFED AVOCADO

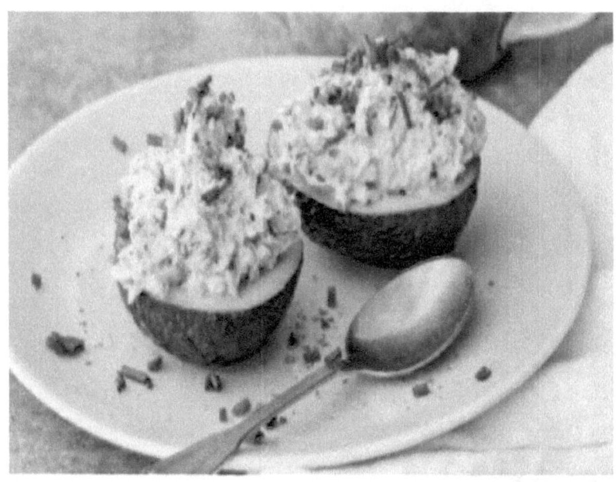

2 Servings

Ingredients

- 1-ounce of red onions (finely chopped)
- One and half ounces of celery stalk (finely chopped)
- Salt and ground black pepper
- One quarter cup of mayonnaise
- 2 avocados (halved lengthwise, pit removed)
- 5 ounces of tuna in water, drained
- 1 table spoon of fresh chives , finely chopped (not compulsory)

Instructions

- ✓ In a mixing bowl, combine the tuna, mayonnaise, celery, and onion. Add the salt and ground black pepper and mix well.
- ✓ Top each half of avocado with an equal amount of tuna filling, then serve with chives on the side.

KETO SHRIMP SKEWERS WITH CHIMICHURRI

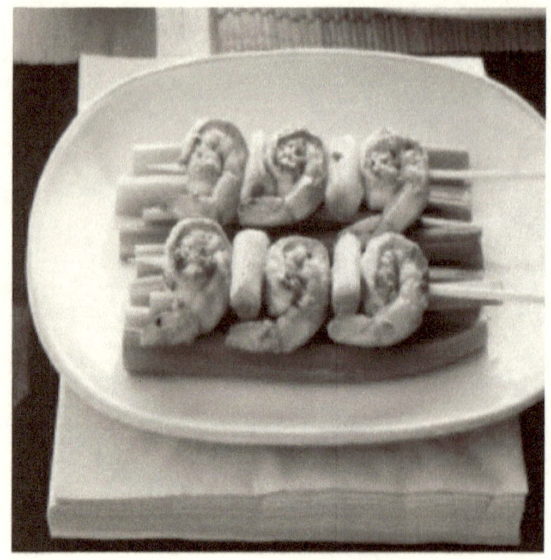

Six servings

Shrimp skewers

- Shrimp (7/4 Ibs)
- 1 lemon juice
- Half teaspoon of salt
- 2 garlic cloves (crushed)
- 1 pinch of chili flakes
- 3 ounces of scallion stalks
- 2 tablespoons of tamari soy sauce

Chimichurri

- One quarter cup of white wine vinegar
- Two ounces of fresh parsley (finely chopped)
- Half cup of light olive oil
- Four garlic cloves (finely chopped)
- Two red chili pepper (finely chopped)
- One pinch of pepper
- One and half teaspoon of salt
- Two teaspoon of dried oregano

Instructions

- ✓ After washing and peeling the shrimp (leaving the tail on it if desired), cut along the top of each shrimp to extract the vein. In a large mixing bowl, combine the lemon juice, soy sauce, crushed garlic, salt, and chili flakes.
- ✓ Add the shrimp to the marinade in the refrigerator and set aside for 15 minutes.
- ✓ Break the green onion stalks into inch-long sticks (2.5cm)

- ✓ While the shrimp are marinating, make the chimichurri. Combine the ingredients in a mixing bowl and stir well, then set aside to allow the flavors to meld.
- ✓ Remove the shrimp from the refrigerator and combine with the other ingredients. Prick the shrimp with wooden kebab sticks, alternating with green onion sticks.
- ✓ Cook the shrimp skewers on a barbacae or gill for about 8 minutes, or until they turn opague.
- ✓ Serve the skewers with chimichurri on the side.

KETO BREAKFAST WITH, TOMATOES FRIED EGG AND CHEESE

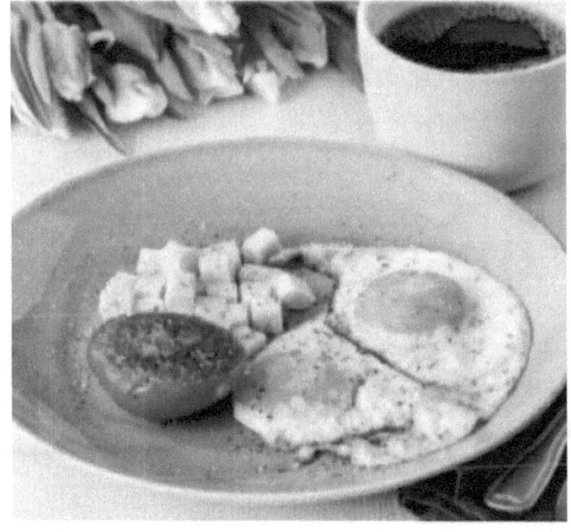

Ingredients:

- Half tablespoon of butter
- 2 ounces of cheddar cheese(cubed)

- 2 eggs
- Salt and ground pepper to season
- Half spoon of dried oregano(not compulsory)
- 2 ounces of tomatoes

Instructions

- ✓ In a frying pan, melt the butter over medium heat.
- ✓ Season the cut sides of the tomatoes with salt and pepper. Place the tomatoes in a frying pan, cut side down.
- ✓ The eggs are cracked into the same frying pan. Enable one side of the egg to fry for sunny side up. For eggs cooked over quick, switch the eggs after a few minutes and cook for another few minutes. Cook for a few minutes longer for firmer yolks, then season with salt and pepper.
- ✓ On a tray, arrange the eggs, onions, and cheese. Serve by sprinkling dried oregano over the eggs and tomatoes to add color and flavor.

KETO BEEF SALAD WITH MOZZARELLA AND TOMATOES

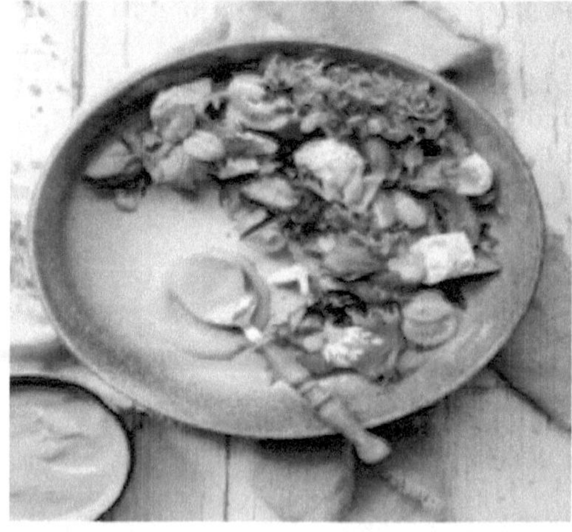

Six servings

Ingredients

Steak

- 1 garlic cloves(minced)

- Salt and pepper to taste
- 2 tablespoons of olive oil
- Sirloin steak at room temperature(2lbs)

Salad

- 11 ounces of mozzarella, mini cheese balls
- Five ounces of leafy greens
- Eleven ounces of multi-colored cheery tomatoes(halved)

Dressing

- 1 tablespoon of fresh basil
- Half tablespoon of fresh oregano
- Two tablespoons of fresh parleys
- One quarter teaspoon of ground black pepper
- Half teaspoon of salt
- Two tablespoons of Dijon mustard
- Three tablespoons of cider vinegar
- Three quarter cups of extra virgin olive oil

Instructions

- ✓ Preheat a large nonstick skillet on the stovetop or an outdoor grill over medium-high heat.
- ✓ Season the steak with salt and pepper. In a cup, mix the olive oil and garlic and rub it all over the steak.
- ✓ Sear the steak for about 5 minutes on either side for a medium rare steak.
- ✓ Remove from the sun, cover loosely with foil, and set aside for 5 minutes.

Salad dressing

- ✓ Hold the mixed greens, cherry tomatoes, and mozzarella on top of a big serving dish. To mix, toss all together.

Garnishing

- ✓ Thinly slice the beef and toss it with other salad ingredients.
- ✓ Add a sprinkling of dressing and freshly cracked black pepper to

finish.

KETO BACON CHEDDAR CORNBREAD WAFFLES WITH EGG AND BACON

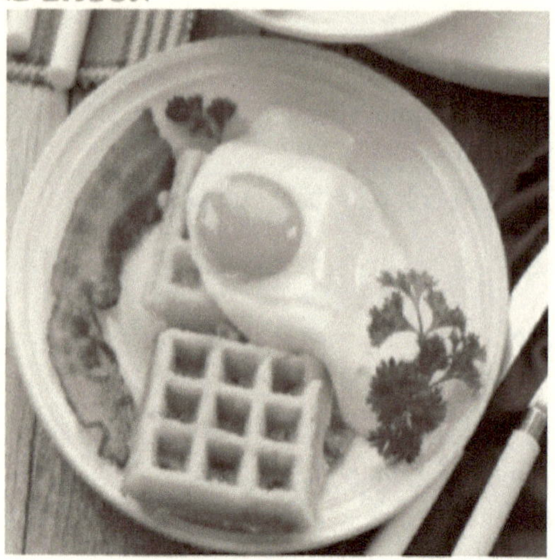

8 servings

Ingredients

- One quarter teaspoon of salt
- 4 ounces of butter(melted)
- One and half teaspoon of baking powder
- One quarter cup of coconut flour (3/4 oz.)
- One third cup of oat fiber
- One third cup of unflavored whey protein isolate
- One quarter cup of water
- 4 eggs
- 4 ounces of cooked bacon(chopped)
- 2 scallions, chopped (1 oz.)
- Half cup of cheddar cheese (2 oz.)
- Half teaspoon of corn extract(not compulsory)
- One third cup of refined coconut oil(melted)

Instructions

✓ Prepare the waffle iron according to the manufacturer's

instructions.

✓ Combine the ingredients in a mixing dish.

✓ Combine the melted butter, eggs, coconut oil, and water in a mixing bowl.

✓ Using a hand mixer, whisk it together.

✓ In the waffle iron, stir together the corn extract, cheese, scallions, and bacon by hand. Scoop the mixture into the wells, being careful not to overfill them.

✓ Cook the waffles until they are browned and crispy, then serve them hot.

KETO HARVEST PUMPKIN SAUSAGE SOUP

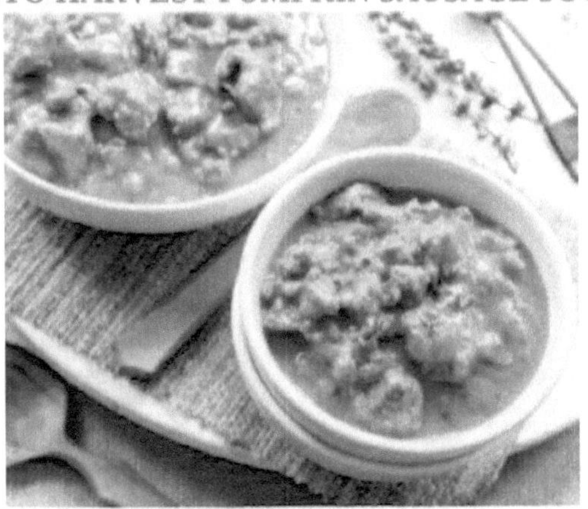

Four servings

Ingredients

- Fresh sausage (3/ 2 lbs)
- 1 pinch of salt
- Half cup of pumpkin puree or crushed tomatoes
- Half teaspoon of red chili pepper flakes (not compulsory)
- Half teaspoon of dried thyme
- 1 tablespoon of salted water
- Half cup of heavy whipping cream
- 1 garlic glove (minced)
- 5 ounces of small red pepper (diced)
- One third cup of white onions (minced)

- One and half cups of chicken broth
- Half teaspoon of rubbed dried sage

Instructions

✓ Brown the sausage, cabbage, onion, and pepper in a broad skillet over medium-high heat.

✓ Drizzle in the seasonings and swirl to blend after the onion and pepper have been browned for up to 15 minutes and the pork has been thoroughly cooked.

✓ Stir in the pumpkin, broth, and cream for 15 to 20 minutes, then will the heat to low and continue to cook, uncovered, until the soup thickens.

✓ Pour in the water, mix well, and serve slightly warm.

KETO BUTTER-FRIED FISH WITH TANDOORI SAUCE

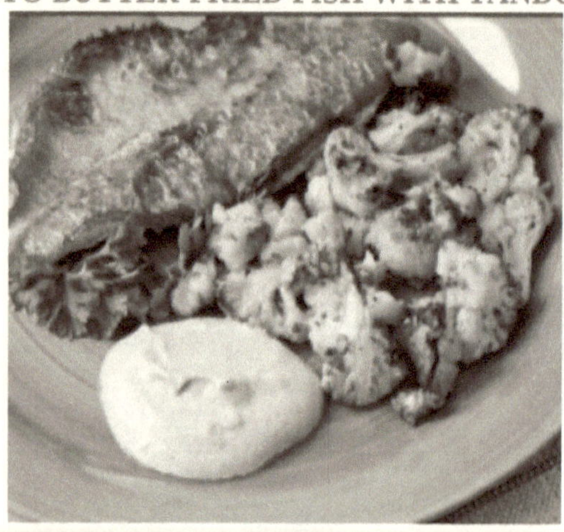

4 servings

Ingredients

- 2 tablespoons of tandoori seasonings
- 2 ounces of butter
- Salt and pepper to taste
- 2 tablespoons of fresh parsley for serving(not compulsory)
- One and half cups of crème fraiche or sour cream
- Cauliflower cut in small florets (1Ibs)

- Boneless fillets or any white fish with skin on(3/2 Ibs)

Instructions

✓ Preheat the oven to 430 degrees Fahrenheit (225 degrees Celsius).

✓ Combine crème fraiche and tandoori seasonings in a mixing bowl, season with salt and pepper to taste, and set aside.

✓ Cauliflower can be divided into small florets or finely sliced into smaller pieces. Sprinkle olive oil over the cauliflower in an ovenproof bowl.

✓ Season with salt and taste. Bake for over 15 minutes in the oven, or until golden brown.

✓ Season the fish on both sides with salt and pepper. Fry skin side down in butter on a high medium high heat. Flip after a few minutes and lower the heat.

✓ Spread some butter on the top side of the fish. The skin should be clean, and the meat should be white.

✓ Garnish with parsley and serve the fish with cauliflower and tandoori sauce.

SPICY SHRIMP SALAD

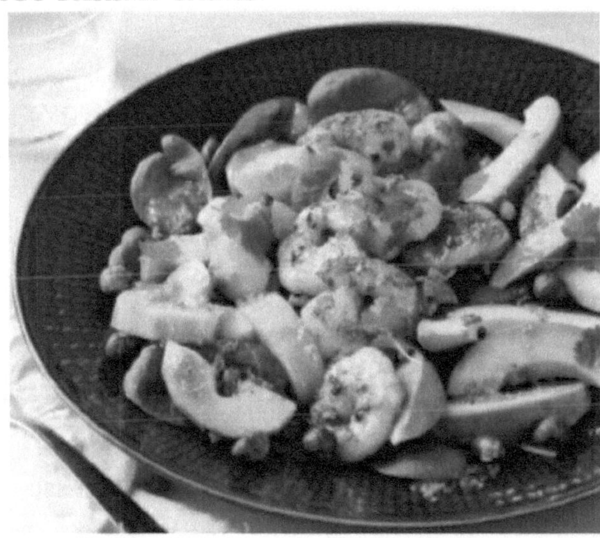

2 servings

- Two (14 oz.) avocados
- Fresh cilantro(for serving)
- Two tablespoons of hazelnuts or salted peanuts(not compulsory)
- For ginger dressing
- One quarter cup of light olive oil or avocado oil
- One tablespoon of fresh ginger (minced)
- Half lime juice
- Five ounces of cucumber
- Two ounces(2 cups) of baby spinach
- Three tablespoons of olive oil (for frying)
- Half tablespoon tamari soy sauce
- Half garlic clove(pressed)
- Salt and pepper to taste
- One garlic glove (pressed)
- Two tablespoons of chili powder or sambal oelek
- Ten ounces of shrimp(peeled)
- Half lime juice

Instructions

✓ Remove the pit from the avocados and cut them in half. Using a spoon, scoop out the avocado pieces and slice them. Squeeze some lime juice over the avocado. After peeling the cucumber, cut it into slices.

✓ Combine spinach, avocado, and cucumber on a plate. Season with salt and pepper.

✓ Fry the garlic and chili in the oil. If the shrimp is not cooked, put it in the pan and fry it for a few minutes on each side. Heat the precooked shrimp quickly and season to taste with salt and pepper.

✓ Attach the shrimp to the vegetables and top with nuts and cilantro.

✓ Combine all of the ingredients in an immersion blender and drizzle over the salad.

Lemon poppy Ricotta Pancakes

Servings: 2 servings

Nutritional content per serving:
Calories-369, fat-25g, protein-29g, Total carbs-6g, fiber-1g, Net carbs-5g

Prep time: 8 minutes

Cook time: 25 minutes

Ingredients

- 1 big lemon (juiced and zested)
- 3 large eggs
- 6 oz. whole milk ricotta
- ¼ cup of almond milk
- 10-12 drops of liquid stevia
- Poppy seeds (1 tablespoon)
- 1 scoop of egg white protein powder
- ¼ cup of powdered erythritol
- ¾ teaspoons of baking powder
- 1 tablespoon of heavy cream

Directions

✓ In a food processor, combine the eggs, ricotta and liquid stevia with half lemon juice and lemon zest. Blend very well and pour into a bowl.

✓ Whisk in the protein powder, almond flour, baking powder, poppy seeds and a pinch of salt.

✓ Heat a big nonstick pan over a medium heat, then spoon the batter into the pan. Use a 1/4 cup of batter per each pancake.

✓ Cook the pancakes until bubbles starts to form in the batter surface, then flip to the other side.

✓ Allow pancake to cook until bottom becomes browned, then

transfer to a plate.

- ✓ Repeat this process with the remaining batter.

- ✓ Whisk the heavy cream, erythrotol powder, reserved lemon zest and juice together.

- ✓ Serve the pancakes hot, with lemon glaze drizzled on it.

Sweet Blueberry Coconut Porridge

Servings: 2 servings

Nutritional content per serving:
Calories-389, Fat-23g, protein-11g, total carbs-39g, fiber-23g, net carbs-16g

Prep time: 8 minutes

Cook time: 20 minutes

Ingredients

- 1 cup of unsweetened almond milk

- ¼ cup of coconut flour

- ¼ cup of canned coconut milk

- 1 tsp of ground cinnamon

- ¼ cup of ground flaxseed

- ¼ tsp of ground nutmeg

- A pinch of salt

- 60g of fresh blue berries

- ¼ cup of shaved coconut.

Directions

- ✓ Place a saucepan over medium heat and warm the coconut milk and almond milk.

✓ Whisk in the flaxseed, coconut oil, nutmeg, Cinnamon and salt into it.

✓ Increase heat and cook until the mixture bubbles.

✓ Then stir in the vanilla extract and sweetener, cook until thickened to your desired level.

✓ Spoon into 2 safe bowls and top with shaved coconut and blue berries

Chorizo Breakfast Bake

Servings: 2 servings

Nutritional content per serving:
Calories-452, Fat-35g, Protein:26g, Total Carbs-5g, Fiber-2g, Net carbs-3g

Prep time: 11 minutes

Cook time: 13 minutes

Ingredients

- 4 oz. chorizo sausage
- 1 tablespoon of extra virgin olive oil
- ½ cup of diced yellow onion
- ½ cup of diced red onion
- 2 large eggs
- 2 slices of thick cut bacon(cooked)
- Salt and pepper

Directions

✓ Preheat oven to 352°F and grease lightly the 2 ramekins.

✓ Heat oil over medium high heat, add onions and pepper and cook for 3-5 minutes until all are browned.

✓ Divide vegetable mixture equally between the 2 ramekins.

- ✓ Chop the chorizo and also divide between the ramekins.

- ✓ Crack an egg into each of the ramekins, seasoning with salt and pepper.

- ✓ Bake for 9-12 minutes until the egg is set to your desired level.

- ✓ Top with the crumbled bacon and serve hot.

Baked Eggs in Avocado

Servings: 1 serving

Nutritional content per serving:

Calories-609, Fat-55g, Protein-21g, Total carbs-17g, Fiber-13g, Net carbs-5g

Prep time: 6 minutes

Cook time: 13-15 minutes

Ingredients

- Lime juice (2 tablespoons)

- 1 medium avocado

- Salt and pepper

- 2 large eggs

- Shredded cheddar cheese (2 tablespoons)

Directions

- ✓ Preheat oven to 440°F

- ✓ Cut avocado into half

- ✓ Scoop out some flesh from the middle of each avocado half

- ✓ Into a baking sheet, Place the avocado halves in an upright position and brush with the lime juice

- ✓ Crack an egg into each half, season to taste with salt and pepper.

- ✓   Bake for 12minutes, then sprinkle cheese on it.

- ✓   Allow the eggs to bake for another 2-3 minutes or until the cheese starts to melt.

- ✓   Serve it hot.

Servings: 1 servings

Nutritional content:

 Calories-495, Fat-30g, Proteon-48g, Total carbs-11g, Fiber-4g, Net carbs-8g

Prep time: 8 minutes

Cook time:18 minutes

Ingredients

- 6 oz. ground pork

- 1 tablespoon of extra virgin oil

- 1/4 cup of diced yellow onion

- 2 tablespoons of diced celery

- ¼ teaspoon of garlic powder

- ¼ teaspoon of onion powder

- 2 tablespoons of soy sauce

- 1 teaspoon of sesame oil

- 1 tablespoon of toasted sesame seeds

- 4 leaves of butter lettuce (separated)

Directions

- ✓   Heat the oil in a skillet placed over medium heat.

- ✓   Add onions, celery, salt, pepper and sauté for 6 minutes until a bit tender.

✓ Stir in the pork and cook until a browned color is formed.

✓ Add onion and garlic powder, then stir in sesame oil and soy sauce.

✓ Add salt and pepper, then remove from heat.

✓ Place the lettuce leaves on a plate, spoon in the pork mixture into them evenly.

✓ To serve, sprinkle with sesame se

Easy Beef Curry

Servings: 3 servings

Nutritional content per serving:

Calories-549, Fat-35g, Protein-49g, Total carbs-15g, Fiber-5.5g, Net carbs-9.5

Prep time: 23 minutes

Cook time: 45 minutes

Ingredients

- 1 medium sized yellow onion(chopped)
- Minced garlic (1 tablespoon)
- Grated ginger (1 tablespoon)
- 1lb beef chunk(chopped)
- 1 ½ cups of canned coconut milk
- Curry powder (2 tablespoons)
- 1 tsp salt
- ½ cup of freshly chopped cilantro

Directions

✓ In a food Processor, combine the garlic, ginger and onion. Blend into a paste.

✓ Transfer the paste into a saucepan and cook for 4 minutes on medium heat.

✓ Stir in coconut milk and gently simmer for 10 minutes.

✓ Add the chopped beef together with salt and curry powder.

✓ Stir, simmer and keep covered for 20minutes.

✓ Remove the lid, simmer for another 20-25 minutes until the beef is well cooked.

✓ Garnish with the freshly chopped cilantro and serve.

Spiced Pumpkin Soup

Servings: 3 servings

Nutritional content per serving:
Caloroes-254, Fat-25g, Protein-11g, Total carbs-9g, Fiber-3g, Net carbs-7g

Prep time: 12 minutes

Cook time: 45 minutes

Ingredients

- 2 tablespoons of butter
- 1 cup of chicken broth
- 1 medium sized onion (chopped)
- ¼ cup of heavy cream
- 3 slices of thick-cut bacon
- Salt and pepper
- 2 cloves of garlic (minced)
- ½ teaspoon of ground cinnamon
- ½ cup of pumpkin puree
- ½ teaspoon of ground nutmeg

Directions

✓ Place a saucepan over medium heat and melt your butter

✓ Add onions, ginger, garlic and cook for 3-5minutes or until onions are translucent

✓　Stir in spices and cook for 2 minutes until fragrant. Season with salt and pepper.

✓　Add the chicken broth and pumpkin. Puree, then bring to a boil.

✓　Reduce heat, Simmer for 25 minutes, then remove from the heat.

✓　Using an immersion blender, puree the soup, then put back to heat, simmer for about 20 minutes.

✓　Cook the bacon until crisp, then put in paper towels for the dressing.

✓　Add the bacon fat and heavy cream into the soup.

✓　Top with the crumbled bacon and serve.

Avocado lime salmon

Servings: 2 servings

Nutritional content per serving:
Calories-568, Fat-45g, Protein-35g, Total carbs-13g, Fiber-9g, Net carbs-4g

Prep time: 14 minutes

Cook time:15 minutes

Ingredients

- 1 big avocado

- Chopped cauliflower (100g)

- Fresh lime juice (1 tablespoon)

- Diced red onion (2 tablespoons)

- 6 oz. boneless salmon fillets

- Salt and pepper

Directions

✓ Put the cauliflower into a food processor and pulse into rice-like grains.

✓ Use cooking spray to grease the skillet and heat over medium heat

✓ Add the cauliflower rice and cook it covered for 7 minutes or until tender. Then set aside.

✓ Again, in a food processor, combine avocado, red onion and lime juice, then blend all smoothly.

✓ In a large skillet over medium heat, put the salmon (skin-side down) and season to taste with salt and pepper.

✓ Cook for 3 to 4 minutes or until seared, change or flip to the other side and cook for additional 3-4 minutes

✓ Serve salmon over a bed of cauliflower rice, top with the avocado cream.

Rosemary Roasted Chicken and Veggies

Servings: 2 servings

Nutritional content per serving:
Calories-538, Fat-40g, Protein-32g, Total carbs-11g, Fiber-3g, Net carbs-8g

Prep time: 12 minutes

Cook time: 38 minutes

Ingredients

- 5 chicken thighs (deboned)

- 1 small sized zucchini (sliced)

- Salt and pepper

- 1 small sized parsnip (peeled and sliced)

- 2 small sized carrots (peeled and sliced)

- 3 tablespoons of extra virgin oil

- 2 cloves of garlic (sliced)

- 1 tablespoon of balsamic vinegar

- 2 teaspoons of freshly chopped rosemary

Directions

✓ Preheat oven to 355°F, grease a small rimmed baking sheet lightly with cooking spray.

✓ Place your chicken thigh on the baking sheet and season with salt and pepper to taste.

✓ Then arrange the veggies and the chicken and sprinkle with the sliced garlic.

✓ Whisk the remaining ingredients together, drizzle them over the chicken and veggies.

✓ Bake for 32 minutes, then broil for about 3-6minutes or until skin is crisp.

Cheesy sausage and mushroom skillet

Servings: 2 servings

Prep time:15 minutes

Cook time: 17 minutes

Ingredients

- Coconut oil (1 tablespoon)

- 6oz Italian sausage (crumbled)

- 4 oz. mushroom (sliced)

- Salt and pepper

- 1 small yellow onion(chopped)

- Dried oregano (1/2 teaspoon)

- Marinara sauce (1/4 cup)

- ¼ cup of water

- Shredded mozzarella

✓ Over medium heat, Preheat oven to 352°F

✓ Place a big cast-iron skillet, heat the oil until it starts smoking.

✓ Add in sausages and cook until it becomes browned and partially cooked.

✓ Then place the sausages on a cutting board and allow it to cool for some minutes.

✓ Add the onion and mushroom into the skillet,cook for 2-4minutes until it turns brown.

✓ Gently slice the sausages and put them back to the skillet.

✓ Stir in the thyme, oregano, salt and pepper.

✓ Pour in the sauce and water, stir very well. Place the skillet over medium heat and cook for 11 minutes.

✓ Sprinkle mozzarella on it and cook for more 3 minutes or until it melts.

Lamb Chops with Rosemary and Garlic

Servings: 1 serving

Nutritional content:

Calories-684, fat-54g, protein-50g, total carbs-7g, fiber-2g, net carbs-5

Prep time:40 minutes

Cook time: 25 minutes

Ingredients

- Melted coconut oil (1 tablespoon)

- Freshly chopped rosemary (1 tablespoon)

- 1 clove garlic (minced)

- 2 bone-in-lamb chops (about 6 oz. meat)

- 1 tablespoon of butter

- 1 tablespoon of extra virgin olive oil

- Salt and pepper

- ¼ lb. fresh asparagus (trimmed)

Directions

✓ In a shallow dish, combine coconut oil, rosemary and garlic together.

✓ Add the lamb chops and turn to coat

✓ Put in the fridge and allow marinate overnight.

✓ Allow the lamb rest at a room temperature for about 30 minutes.

✓ Place a large skillet over medium-high heat.

✓ Add lamp chops, cook for 5minutes, then season to taste with salt and pepper.

✓ Turn the other side of the chops and cook for additional 5 minutes or until it is cooked to your desired level.

✓ Allow lamb chops to rest for 5minutes before serving.

✓ Meanwhile, use olive oil, pepper and salt to toss the asparagus.

✓ Then spread asparagus on a baking sheet.

✓ Broil for 8-10 minutes until it becomes charred, shake it occasionally.

✓ Serve it hot together with the lamb chops.

Fat-Busting Vanilla Protein Smoothies

Nutritional content:
 Calories-549, Fat-45g, Protein-24g, Total carbs-7g, Fiber-0.4g, Net carbs-6.6

Servings:1 serving

Prep time-6 minutes

Cook time-0 minutes

Ingredients

- heavy cream (1/2 cup)
- 20g or 1 scoop of vanilla egg white protein powder.
- 5 ice cubes
- 1/4 cup of vanilla almond milk
- 1 tablespoon of erythritol powder
- 1 teaspoon of coconut oil
- 1/4 cup of whipped cream
- 1/4 teaspoon of vanilla extract

Directions

- ✓ In a blender, combine all ingredients except the whipped cream.
- ✓ Blend for 35-60seconds or until thoroughly smooth.
- ✓ Pour contents into a glass and top it with the whipped cream.

Pepper Jack Sausage Egg Muffins
Servings: 3 servings

Nutritional content per serving:
 Calories-454, Fat-36g, Protein-25g, Total carbs-3g, Fiber-1g, Net Carbs-2g

Prep time: 8 minutes

Cook time: 35 minutes

Ingredients

- 10 oz. of breakfast sausage(ground)

- ¼ teaspoon of garlic powder

- ¼ cup of diced yellow onion

- 3 large eggs (whisked)

- Salt and pepper

- ½ cup of shredded pepper jack cheese

- Heavy cream (2 tablespoons).

Directions

✓ Preheat oven to 348°F, then grease 3 ramekins with a cooking spray.

✓ Stir ground sausage, garlic powder, diced onion, salt and pepper together in a mixing bowl.

✓ Divide the mixture of sausage equally in the ramekins, press them into the bottom and sides, leave only the middle open.

✓ Whisk eggs, heavy cream, salt and pepper together in a mixing bowl.

✓ Divide egg mixture among sausage cups and top it with shredded cheese.

✓ Bake for 30-35minutes or until the eggs are set and cheese is browned.

Mozzarella Veggies-Loaded Quiche

Servings: 1 serving

Nutritional Content:

Calories-589, Fat-41g, Protein-37g, Total carbs-25g, Fiber-7g, Net carbs-18g

Prep time: 9 minutes

Cook time: 27 minutes

Ingredients

- 1 tablespoon of grated Parmesan cheese
- 2 large eggs
- 6 tablespoons of almond flour
- 1/4 cup of frozen spinach (thawed and drained)
- 1/4 cup of zucchini
- 1/4 cup of shredded mozzarella cheese
- 1 tablespoon of heavy cream
- 4 cherry tomatoes (halved)
- Heavy cream (1 tablespoon)
- Chopped chives (1 teaspoon)

Directions

✓ In a bowl, stir together almond flour, grated Parmesan, 1 egg and a pinch of salt, do not stop stirring until a soft dough is formed.

✓ Press the dough into the bottom of a small pan, as evenly as possible.

✓ Score the dough's sides and bottom, bake for 8 minutes at 324°F and allow to cool.

✓ In a skillet, cook the bacon until its color changes to brown, crumble and spread it in a quiche pan.

✓ Sprinkle in zucchini, spinach, cheese and tomatoes.

✓ Whisk the remaining egg together with heavy cream, chives, salt and pepper. Pour into the quiche.

✓ Bake for 20-25 minutes until eggs are set.

✓ Serve hot and enjoy.

Pan-Fried Pepperoni Pizzas

Servings: 3 servings

Nutritional content per serving:
 Calories-546, Fat-43g, Protein-33g, Total carbs:13g, Fiber-7g, Net Carbs-6g.

Prep time:8 minutes

Cook time:30 minutes

Ingredients

- 6 tablespoons of grated Parmesan cheese.

- Extra virgin olive oil (3 tablespoons)

- 6 large eggs

- Psyllium husk powder (3 tablespoons)

- 5 oz. of shredded mozzarella (Divided)

- 2 oz. of dried pepperoni (divided)

- 2 teaspoons of Italian seasoning

- Fresh chopped basil (3 tablespoons) .

Directions

✓ In a blender, combine eggs, psyllium husk powder, Parmesan, Italian seasoning and a pinch of salt.

✓ Blend until it becomes thoroughly smooth. Rest for 6 minutes.

✓ . In a skillet over medium heat, heat a tablespoon of extra virgin olive oil.

✓   Spoon in 1/3rd of batter into the skillet, spread it into a circle, cook until it becomes brown underneath.

✓   Flip the pizza crust, cook until the other side becomes brown.

✓   Transfer crust to a foil line baking sheet and repeat this process with the remaining batter.

✓   Spoon in 3-tanlespoon of the low carb tomato sauce over each of the crust.

✓   Top with shredded cheese and diced pepperoni, broil until the cheese is browned.

✓   Sprinkle with the fresh basil, slice pizza and serve.

Savory **Ham and Cheese Waffles**
Servings: 2 servings

Nutritional content per serving:
Calories-570, Fat-46g, Protein-34g, Total carbs-4g, Fiber-0g, Net carbs-4g

Prep time: 12 minutes

Cook time:30 minutes

Ingredients

- 4 large eggs (Divided)

- 1/3 cup of melted butter

- 40g or 2 scoop of egg white's protein powder

- ½ teaspoon of salt

- 1 oz. of dried ham

- ¼ cup of shredded cheddar cheese.

- 1 teaspoon of baking powder.

Directions

✓ Separate the 2 eggs and set aside

✓ Beat the 2 egg yolks with the protein powder, butter, baking powder and salt in a mixing bowl.

✓ Fold in chopped ham and the cheddar cheese.

✓ In a separate bowl, whisk in the egg whites, add a pinch of salt until the stiff peaks starts forming.

✓ Fold the beaten egg whites in the egg yolk mixture. Make this in 2 batches.

✓ Grease the preheated waffle maker, spoon in 1/4 cup of batter into it and close.

✓ Cook until the waffle turns to a golden brown color, about 4-5minutes, then remove.

✓ Repeat this process with the remaining batter.

✓ Meanwhile, in the skillet, heat oil and fry your eggs with salt and pepper.

✓ Serve the waffle hot, topped with a fried egg.

Keto Friendly Snacks

You might feel hungry within the day, it's advisable you have some keto-friendly snacks ready. These keto-friendly snacks are ever ready to help you:

1. **Nuts:** pecans, Brazil nuts, macadamias, walnuts.

2. **Pork rinds**

3. **Seeds**: Pumpkin, chia, flax, sunflower etc.

4. **Guacamole**- carrots, celery, peppers, dip pork rinds or any of your favorite low- carb vegetable.

5. **Avocados**

6. **But butters**: Almond, peanut, coconut, cashew etc. Do not add any sugar.

7. Pickles

8. Jerky

9. Seaweed

10. Quest bars

Common Allergens

To make this meal plan easy for you, here are most common food allergens and what you can use to substitute them:

- **Eggs:** replace an egg with 2 1/2 tablespoons of flax or chia seed which has already been soaked for 5 minutes in 3 tbps of water.

- **Coconut:** You may replace coconut oil with butter or other oil types in the ratio of 1:1

- **1/4 coconut flour** may also be replaced with 1 cup of almond flour.

- **Shellfish:** Shellfishes such as shrimp may be replaced with any meat you like eating.

- **Nuts:** Pumpkin seeds, sunflower seeds, flax or chia seeds may be used in place of nuts.

- Seed butter or tahini may be used in place of but butters.

- **Diary**: coconut cream may be used in place of heavy cream in the ratio of 1:1.

- **Coconut oil** may be used to replace butter in the ratio of 1:1

- **Mayonnaise** may be replaced with sour cream and cream cheese in the ratio of 1:1

- **Diary yoghurt** may be replaced with unsweetened coconut milk oil in the ratio of 1:1.

Conclusion

This keto diet meal plan is organized specifically for you as it shows delicious and easy diet that will give you the perfect body shape and boost your self-confidence. If you adhere strictly to this meal plan, you will notice a lot of positive changes in your body just within 21 days or 3 weeks. Try your best to keep to it, it will give you all what you are looking for in your body.

www.ingramcontent.com/pod-product-compliance
Lightning Source LLC
Chambersburg PA
CBHW020944160726
47993CB00007B/2935